The Lemon Detox Diet

Rejuvenation Sensation

The Lemon Detox Diet

Rejuvenation Sensation

Dr K A Beyer

pnp

Published by PNP Ltd
P.O. Box 6554
Grantham
Lincs NG32 3FE

ISBN-10   0 9553229 0 1
ISBN-13   978 0 9553229 0 7

CAUTION

If you have a medical condition, or are pregnant or diabetic
Type 1, the detox programme described in this book should not
be followed without first consulting your doctor or practitioner.
All guidelines and warnings should be read carefully, and the
author and publisher cannot accept responsibility for injury
arising out of a failure to comply with the same.

Printed in Great Britain by Creative Print and Design Group

Contents

Preface

The Lemon Detox Diet Rejuvenation Sensation is a ten-day holistic naturopathic journey to better health: simple, enjoyable and totally natural.

Amazingly effective, this cleansing programme will rid your body of accumulated toxins and help you to lose excess weight.

During the programme, we replace solid food with a Natural Tree Syrup & lemon drink: a natural beverage of tree syrups, pure lemon juice, water and cayenne pepper carefully formulated to provide nourishment while supporting the body as it cleanses itself.

The Lemon Detox Diet works by stimulating your body's own natural cleansing process by giving it a break from the constant work of digestion, and allowing balance to be restored.

Some people worry about going without solid foods, but the *The Lemon Detox Diet Rejuvenation Sensation* is a health programme, not a traditional fast. A true fast is complete abstinence from food of any kind, *The Lemon Detox Diet* is a semi-fast programme based on nourishing and energizing liquid food and is carried out for a limited period of time. Its purpose is to purify the body and free the system of excess fats and deposits.

In nature, fasting is a completely natural process. In all major religions of the world it forms an essential part of physical and spiritual cleansing – only in modern times is it believed so firmly that all things should be planned and that man should be programmed in accordance with the scientific knowledge of the moment.

People who have completed the programme report a wide variety of benefits including:

- cleansing the body of toxins
- effective weight loss
- increased vigour and vitality
- better digestion
- sounder sleep
- better circulation
- shiny hair and stronger nails
- clear skin and eyes
- greater resistance to illness
- reduced dependence on supplements and drugs
- fortified will-power and determination
- improved concentration and clarity of thought
- balanced emotions
- happier, more positive outlook
- sense of inner peace.

The Lemon Detox Diet is for anyone who feels the need to take a more conscious control of their life. It is a commitment towards bringing out the best in ourselves; towards exploring our potential and living life to the full.

1: Introduction

I would like to introduce you to an amazingly effective naturopathic detox programme that will help you to cleanse your body of accumulated toxins and will also help you to lose excess weight. It's natural, simple and safe.

Originally created by the legendary Hawaiian naturopath Stanley Burroughs as a cure for stomach ulcers, it was later refined in Switzerland into its present form as a detox programme.

The programme now has a huge following around the world, where it is known by several names: *The Lemon Detox Diet* in the UK and Eire; *Neera Supercleanse* in the USA; *The Rejuvenation Sensation* in Australia, *Le Regime Vital* in France and *La Cura de Savia y Zumo de Limon* in Spain.

In this book you will find precise instructions on how to follow *The Lemon Detox Diet*, together with some of the principle ideas of Stanley Burroughs, from his book *Healing For The Age Of Enlightenment*. Above all, you will see how this process has developed as a treatment of purification. We shall only be quoting a few of the successes achieved, because the many testimonies would exceed the limitations of this book.

The Lemon Detox Diet is ideal for detoxification and also as a kick-start for weight loss management and a means of training the appetite – but only personal experience will show you what the diet is capable of achieving in each individual case. Most people turn to this diet to cleanse the system, to lose weight or to help gain relief from a digestive problem or medical complaint.

The following pages will deal firstly with the practical aspects of the programme, followed by precise instructions on how to carry it out. In chapters 12 and 13 we briefly present the opinions of Stanley Burroughs (the creator of this method) on health and illness, conventional medicine and naturopathic medicine.

And at the end of this book there is a small chapter with many letters of thanks that testify to the effectiveness of the *The Lemon Detox Diet*. But remember, only personal experience can show what the diet is capable of achieving in each individual case.

Word of the diet spreads

The success of *The Lemon Detox Diet* can be seen from its popular use among doctors and naturopaths. The observations of health professionals can be read in chapter 14, which gives useful advice for all those trying the programme for the first time.

In the French clinics of the acclaimed homoeopath/naturopath and author – Dr Catherine Kousmine – *Le Regime Vital* (as *The Lemon Detox Diet* is known in France), is used in numerous cases as a basic preparatory treatment to retrain the appetite prior to introducing new healthier eating habits.

Without any doubt, a body that is healthy and purified will respond more favourably to any positive change and produce the rebirth of the innate intelligence of our organism. **Dr Catherine Kousmine**

In England, Dr Michel Odent – the obstetrician who pioneered natural childbirth and birthing pools in UK hospitals – uses the detox programme as part of his recently developed *Accordion Method,* a pre-conception programme to help parents to have healthier babies.

The duration of each session is about four days. During day two and day three of such a session there is no food available other than a specially designed cocktail made from a mixture palm tree syrup, maple syrup and lemon juice. Cayenne pepper is added after dilution (a way to slightly increase the body temperature and therefore sweat excretion). The cocktail can be consumed at any time without any restriction. It makes the fasting period comfortable. Its mineral content is exceptionally rich. The ratio of zinc to man-

ganese to iron is ideal (in the region of 5:2:1). The ratio of calcium to magnesium is around 2.5:1, and the ratio of potassium to sodium around 10:1. The lemon juice represents the main source of natural vitamin C. **Dr Michael Odent**

The Lemon Detox Diet is also beneficial to the hair and for aesthetic treatments in general. The Hair Institute of Switzerland makes the programme an obligatory part of their treatment.

Waste products are deposited in the outermost cells of the body, which includes those in the hair. For healthy hair, detoxification of the body is absolutely necessary and to this end nothing is better than this diet. **The Hair Institute, Switzerland**

This revised edition, which has been completed based on experiences in Europe and America, aims remove any prejudices and to leave you full of enthusiasm.

2: Lose 7-12lbs in ten days

Just a simple slogan?

This title causes suspicion. Is it possible? And if so, is it healthy? Is it an exaggerated promise, or a simple publicity slogan? Or is it really possible to lose so much weight with a simple diet of Natural Tree Syrup and lemon juice?

Seven to 12lbs is indeed a substantial amount to lose in just ten days. It is even more amazing that most people regain little (if any) of the weight they have lost weight after the diet. In past tests, 70% of the people who followed the *The Lemon Detox Diet* exactly as described in this book lost between 10-20lbs in ten days, while most of the remaining 30% lost between 6-10lbs. This is even more surprising if you think that not all of those who followed the programme were overweight.

The majority of those who are not overweight lose between 4-6lbs, and those who are underweight reestablish the balance of the body's metabolism. The body regains its natural balance of elements and is better able to maintain its optimum weight after completing the programme.

The fat just dissolves

The fact that one's weight after the diet is maintained, proves that the loss of weight consists not only of loss of water but also of loss of fat. Stanley Burroughs described the phenomenon as if 'the fat dissolves almost literally'. Those doing *The Lemon Detox Diet* can experience it for themselves. Only this way can the great loss of weight be explained. If the body had to burn off all the excess fat, the process would take much longer.

The Lemon Detox Diet is completely safe – the loss of weight is no more than a secondary effect. The principle effect is the detoxification of the organs of the body, and at the same time the body rids itself superfluous fat deposits. Weight loss is a side effect of this purification in the course of which the skin and hair are embellished, digestion is normalized together with the cholesterol level, and diverse corporal irregularities disappear. The purification also affects the psychic state in a positive way, as we will see in chapter 11.

Put it to the test

A practical test is more revealing than thousands of theories. The numerous enthusiastic testimonies weigh more than all the doubts that could be raised against *The Lemon Detox Diet*. Nutritionists have tried in vain to prove that it is not possible to lose so much weight in so little time. All I can reply is that I respect their theories but suggest that they put the programme to the test. There are many who have been convinced.

People often doubt that they are capable of changing their bad habits. Here the programme lends itself to being an almost revolutionary support, as it breaks practically all our bad habits at once. The confidence of being able to change and give up voluntarily our normal habits is an important base on which to build a healthier lifestyle. In many cases the problem of excess weight has its origin in an excess of psychological temptations, in other words, 'I eat because I feel empty inside': a frustration at lack of affection, values of recognition by others, insecurity or nervousness. 'By eating, I am trying to fill this vacuum.'

The programme works not only at a physical level but also purifies, lifts and strengthens at a mental and emotional level: as we know, everything about our being is interrelated.

To be able to solve the problem of excess weight, it is advisable to decide conscientiously while carrying out the diet, to introduce eating and life habits which are healthier, integral and satisfactory; to do some form of sport, walk every day; and try not to react to frustration, anger and bad feeling by eating or drinking anything. It is only then that you can see that you have not only lost weight but you have also lost your bad eating habits.

Many people have found it a great help to keep a diary during the diet, noting down the changes that are occurring daily: how they feel, what they are dreaming of, and above all, the new and better eating habits that they want to introduce into their lives after the detox programme has been completed.

Experience is the mother of science

It is best that you first read this book, paying special attention to chapters 4, 5 and 6. After that you can put it to the test. And although you may not believe it, in ten days you will be lighter, healthier and at the same time will feel marvellous!

During the detox programme, sensitivity towards your surroundings will increase and to a considerable degree your creative and intuitive capacity will also increase.

Make the most of these new horizons that will open up to you. Many people in these first days of the diet open their minds and take pleasure in classical or religious music; spontaneously they discover the beauty of nature, or perceive for the first time an harmonious mental state, peace with oneself and the rest of the universe, self-confidence, and the pleasure of being alive. It is in these moments that problems often lose their importance and a new intuitive perception can become a way towards internal freedom.

For this reason, the best time to carry out the detox programme is when you are not under pressure from work and social commitments, away from the draining stresses and obligations of everyday life.

The detox programme beckons you to reflection, to moments of silence, to finding yourself and to recreational activity.

You will want to retire consciously into your own personal space, do things that you feel like doing, rest whenever your body asks for it, and without hurrying, take pleasure in the new experiences that the detox programme provides.

3: Natural Tree Syrup

What is Natural Tree Syrup?

Natural Tree Syrup, which comes from the saps of the maple tree of northern regions and the Arenga and Kitul palms that grow in the tropics, plays a very important part in *The Lemon Detox Diet*.

At one time, the original diet used only maple syrup. However, through various analyses it was shown that the mineral content in maple syrup is subject to natural variations. Natural growing conditions, such as the quality of the earth, and climatic influences all play a part. Therefore the maple syrup did not have, on its own, consistent levels of the necessary nutrients to keep the dieter healthy for the ten days of the detox programme.

The Lemon Detox Diet demands a highly consistent and balanced mineral content, and after extensive research – of over five years and thousands of tests – it was found that the syrup of several rare Asian palm trees contained the ideal complementary nutrients. So in this way Natural Tree Syrup was created to respond completely to the requirements of the detox programme and the diet.

For our body to function properly, it is important to measure the quantity of minerals that we consume, and to get the right balance between such minerals, as would be found in their natural environment. This also applies to the sugar content. Natural Tree Syrup does not contain any artificial sugar. The presence of glucose is derived 100% from natural palm and maple syrup, which also contains the natural trace elements that are needed for organic assimilation.

Natural Tree Syrup is one of the tastier food products that mother earth provides. It is comprised only of natural food substances – which are concentrated in the palm and maple trees – as they exist in nature.

The importance of lemon

The two principal ingredients of *The Lemon Detox Diet* are fresh lemons and Natural Tree Syrup. The humble lemon, a fruit with an extraordinary number of uses, is one of the main sources of minerals and vitamins and contains the widest range of medicinal properties of all citrus fruits.

The Arab, Greek and Roman doctors knew of its beneficial effects as a cure and preventative measure against illness. It was used in both Ayurvedic and

Chinese traditional medicine, and later adopted by European folk medicine. Today it has an important place in natural treatments and as a natural antiseptic.

The following elements of lemon juice are particularly significant: basic citric acid has a pleasant taste and carries out important functions in the body. It also acts as a preventative to rickets as it is important in the gelling of calcium.

The citric acid cycle is a very important chain of biochemical reactions during the course of which – by means of the metabolism of the cells – the exothermic reaction made of the intermediary product (coenzyme acetylic A), is a result of the metabolism of the proteins, lipids and carbohydrates.

The action of the citric acid allows – through the metabolism of the proteins, lipids and hydro carbonates – the elimination of fatty deposits in the tissues; and from this action we achieve weight loss.

The lack of vitamin C (ascorbic acid), causes an illness by the name of rickets that has been known since the time of the Crusades. Treatment for this ailment by lemon juice has been used since the 18th century.

Vitamin C is indispensable for healthy bones, teeth and blood vessels. This vitamin increases the resistance of the body to infection and is very important for a healthy metabolism. It is necessary for anti-oxidants (substances that stop the breakdown of the cells by oxygen) to work well. During the period of the programme, the daily absorption of lemon juice is more than 80mg (suggested quantity: 75mg per day for an adult), and the body is activated through an improved metabolism. In this way each cell can get rid of the waste and residues, which is why the patient feels very well and in good physical shape during *The Lemon Detox Diet*.

Maple syrup

Maple syrup comes from the vast maple forests of North America where the native Indians were already proficient in the process of extraction of this sweet sap and knew how to prepare and preserve the syrup. As sugar was a rarity in those latitudes, maple syrup became an important basic foodstuff.

The syrup also provided the Indians with an energizing tonic, and during periods of illness they would frequently consume only water and extracts of medicinal plants combined with maple syrup, which increased the curative properties of the plants.

Today, most commercial maple syrup has nothing to do with authentic maple syrup extract. It is only a cheap industrial imitation and it completely lacks the high nutritional and purifying value of the authentic syrup.

The Bird's-Eye Maple, one of over 75 varieties of maple, produces its sweet sap only during a period of four to six weeks in March and April when the temperate spring begins in Canada.

At this time of year the trees are still covered with more than a metre of snow, making the harvest of the sap an arduous and bitter task.

Every morning the sap is collected from containers, which hang from the trees. To be able to preserve the sweet sap, a concentrate is obtained by evaporating the water content. Forty to 50 litres of harvested sap – the quantity that one mature maple tree can produce in a year – are required to obtain just one litre of concentrated syrup. This is equivalent to the quantity which one large maple tree can produce in a year. In addition, the maple tree must be at least 40 years old before it is mature enough to be tapped and the sap extracted, otherwise it would be harmful to the tree.

The harvest of maple syrup can be divided into three phases, recognizable through their colour and denominated grade: A, B & C.

Grade A is obtained from the first phase of the annual harvest, it is the most abundant and contains more sugars and fewer mineral salts. Its colour is a light amber. It is a sweetener with wide application, and is used in commercial confectionary.

Grade B is the middle phase, also very sweet, but slightly darker in colour, and is used in the specialist gourmet market.

Grade C is obtained from the last phase of the

harvest, when the sap is thicker. This grade, the least refined, is of a higher quality, but is not so abundant and is less sweet, and contains a much higher level of mineral salts compared to grades A or B. Grade C maple syrup contains a high level of calcium, zinc, manganese and iron (more than double that of grade A. Its colour is dark amber.

As *The Lemon Detox Diet* requires the maintenance of a balanced high level of minerals, only grade C is used in the Natural Tree Syrup diet mix so as to prevent possible deficiencies.

Palm syrup or Neera

Palm syrup (or Neera) is the primary ingredient of the Madal Bal Natural Tree Syrup. Neera is a Sanskrit word, which roughly translates to palm syrup, but its fuller meaning is 'life essence of the palm tree'. Palm tree syrup was added to the original programme because it was found that it contains many important minerals.

The palm is one of the oldest plants on earth. Among the hundreds of varieties of palm tree that grow in the tropics, three are especially beneficial to man – the coco palm, the oil palm and the sugar palm. In the Northern Hemisphere, there is only one type of maple that produces the sweet syrup; likewise in the tropics there are also only two or three varieties of the sugar palm whose sap can be used to obtain this particular syrup.

As with the maple syrup, the production of palm syrup is equally painstaking. This sap is obtained by cutting the stem of the palm when it is about to flower. The sap falls drop by drop from the cut into a bamboo container. Agile boys rapidly climb up and down the trees twice a day to empty the containers.

Later, the sap is heated in large vessels over an open fire until it thickens and becomes the consistency of syrup. It is then filtered and refined to avoid possible impurities resulting from the primitive form of harvesting. No additives, natural preservatives or other modern chemical forms of preserving are used.

Palm syrup is used only in its place of production and is seldom exported, as it is difficult to store in a warm and humid climate. If it has to be stored, the syrup undergoes concentration to dry sugar to avoid fermentation.

Natural Tree Syrup uses tree syrup from several Southeast Asian palm species, including the Coconut Palm, the Arenga and Kitul Palms of the rainforests, the Nipah Palm of the swamps and marshes and the Palmyra Palm of northern Sri Lanka.

Natural Tree Syrup uses only palm tree syrup produced by small family farms, using techniques introduced and monitored by international aid organizations. This labour intensive form of production is certainly more expensive than large-scale plantation methods, but it ensures the highest quality organic syrup and helps local communities develop by supporting family based enterprise.

Palm syrup and palm sugar are considered to be great delicacies in their own countries and are preferred to white sugar because of their superior taste. Tests show that palm syrup is abundant in minerals – especially potassium and calcium – and therefore ideal for *The Lemon Detox Diet.*

Palm syrup stands out because of its high level of potassium, and for its perfect balance with its counterpart, sodium (10:1).

Maintaining these proportions is of vital importance because potassium is involved in a great number of cellular processes, which would be inhibited by high concentrations of sodium

Conversely, a total lack of sodium would dehydrate the body, a factor that must be taken into account during the detox programme, during which no other food is consumed.

Due to the requirements of the cells there should be about ten times more potassium than calcium, which is exactly the proportion that is found in the mixture of maple and palm syrups.

Natural Tree Syrup:
an ideal combination

Both maple and palm syrup are foodstuffs that are rich in minerals and are complementary to each other.

Analysis Results: (varies due to climate change)

Mineral content	mg per 100g
Iron	2.88
Manganese	1.20
Zinc	2.69
Magnesium	20.3
Calcium	86.8
Sodium	45.7
Copper	0.15
Potassium	395.0

Composition	g per 100g
Water	23.3
Protein	0.56
Fats	0.30
Carbohydrate (fruit sugars)	74.6

Calcium

Calcium is essential for the normal growth of bones and teeth; it helps in the healthy functioning of the muscles and the nerves as well as the circulation of the blood. It helps nerve conditions, muscle contraction, blood clotting and membrane permeability. Clinically, it can be used for preventing or treating osteoporosis in post-menopausal women, reducing blood pressure in hypertensive patients and gives possible protection against colon cancer. The association of citric acid and calcium is very positive.

Iron

Iron is indispensable for all living creatures. Iron is an essential mineral necessary for many important metabolic functions in the body. It is part of haemoglobin, the oxygen-carrying component of the blood. Iron not attached to the haemoglobin in red blood cells is stored in the liver, bone marrow, spleen, and muscles. It has an important relation to the cycle of citric acid (lemon). The most important reason to take iron as a supplement is to alleviate anaemia that is caused by too little iron in the body. People who are deficient in iron are usually pale, have poor circulation, suffer vertigo, melancholia, and have difficulty in concentration.

Manganese

Manganese is an indispensable element as it is a regenerator of carbohydrates, cholesterol, iron and copper. It plays an important part in the skeletal and genital glands development. Essential for all reactions that require adenosine triphosphate (the energy currency of the body cells) it regulates all muscle contractions. It is used in the prevention or treatment of many types of heart disease, it enhances bone formation in sufferers of osteoporosis and improves lung function in asthmatics.

Zinc

Zinc helps with the growth of the body and the skeleton, the regeneration of the skin and the hair cells and activates the scaling process. It also plays an important part in the metabolism of the albumin and assures the normal secretion of insulin. The amount of zinc present in the body is often on the low side, and this can be balanced with grade C maple syrup.

Potassium

The most important functions of potassium are the transmission of nerve impulses, control of skeletal muscle and maintenance of blood pressure. It is essential for protein synthesis and the storage of glycogen. It is used for the prevention and treatment of high blood pressure, diseases associated with malnutrition, gastrointestinal disorders and alkalosis.

Apart form its high and valuable content of mineral salts, vitamins and enzymes, Natural Tree Syrup supplies the body with a high degree of carbohydrates, which are easily assimilated.

Carbohydrates: (Fructose and Glucose)

These constitute an immediate source of energy for the body. The high levels of fructose and glucose in Natural Tree Syrup ensure the necessary support to the body, in particular the nervous system and the brain cells, which essentially depend on glucose as a source of energy.

The Lemon Detox Diet does not produce negative effects such as fatigue, nervousness or lack of energy, which often occur in other types of weight-loss diets that are low in carbohydrates and trace elements. Healthy people do not notice any fatigue or nervousness during the treatment, maintaining a good physical capacity and feelings of perfect well-being.

The reduction of fatty deposits in the body is a desirable side effect of the programme The glucose content of the Natural Tree Syrup and the vitamin C of the lemon protect the liver where numerous vital metabolic reactions are carried out. And detoxification of the liver is speeded up through the treatment. The relationship between the intestines and the liver plays an important part, which is why the daily cleansing of the intestines is absolutely necessary during *The Lemon Detox Diet*.

Palm and maple saps are practically the only sweeteners that are 100% natural; the trees are not cultivated by man, and grow without human intervention, fertilizers are not used, nor are any other methods of modern cultivation employed. They are the only trees in the world to be unharmed by the harvesting of their precious sap.

Some comments about white sugar

White sugar, refined and industrialized, is almost completely lacking in energy when it arrives at our table. As the vitamin and mineral content is 0%, the body needs substances such as calcium, Group B vitamins and proteins in order to absorb it.

Because of this, it is recommended that refined sugar be replaced by natural sweeteners, which not only do not drain the body of the basic substances, but provide minerals, vitamins and enzymes.

An excess of refined and artificial foods could easily be avoided with a more conscious healthy diet. White sugar causes damage to the teeth, intestines and bones.

4: The Lemon Detox Diet: a holistic view

Three basic rules

According to Stanley Burroughs there are three basic rules for a diet that maintains the body in optimum condition for cleansing, recovery and preservation. A body that is ill must first be purified, only then can it recover and preserve its health.

Cleansing

The cleansing process is also the basis of other curative treatments, such as the *Fruit Juice Diet* developed by the Austrian, Herr Rudolf Breuss. Other fasting treatments, which only allow the intake of water, are also directed towards the cleansing of the body. The disadvantage of total fasting is that the body loses all its minerals and vitality. Total fasting is only recommended when the body has been receiving a full diet of nutrients for a protracted period of time. A diet based on fruit juices allows the body to both rest and detoxify, providing only the essential nutrients.

Regenerating the body

The main purpose of the programme is the detoxification of the body, dissolving and eliminating accumulated impurities. It cleans and decongests the digestive tract, and the other organs such as the liver and kidneys. Blood pressure is regulated, and this helps to produce good circulation. In this way it is possible to achieve a youthful appearance and greater elasticity of the body, whatever your age.

All catarrh related illnesses, such as the common cold, flu, fevers, sinusitis and bronchitis are quickly improved or even eliminated, freeing the individual of various allergies that form the basis of later respiratory difficulties and obstruction of the sinuses. The allergies are often a result of the accumulation of toxins, which disappear with the purging of the body.

Illnesses that are a result of calciferous deposits in the joints, muscles, cells and glands, are easily improved and in some cases resolved. The cholesterol deposits in the arteries and veins drop quite dramatically through the miraculous purification of *The Lemon Detox Diet*.

Skin infections disappear when the rest of the body

is cleansed. Boils, abscesses and spots… these eruptions are nature's way of quickly eliminating poisons from the body.

All types of infection are the result of accumulations of poisons that are dissolved, burned or oxidized in order to purify the body. For this reason, the required rapid elimination of the toxins give rise to infectious fevers. Infections are not 'caught', they are created by nature in order to help with the burning of the remains of waste products.

However, the *The Lemon Detox Diet* is not directed to one particular form of illness, but gives the body the space to recover, purify, regenerate and increase its defences. In other words it deals with a cleansing treatment of diverse uses that can also be applied as a preventative measure, for example in the case of a wave of colds, a flu epidemic (see chapter 13), or other more dangerous illnesses.

The majority of illnesses originate in the digestive system, which is often overloaded; food is not well digested and waste products and toxins accumulate. By means of *The Lemon Detox Diet* the load is lightened, and by maintaining a healthy light diet we are able to maintain a healthy digestive tract even after the programme is finished.

Excess weight loss is probably the most common side effect of the detox programme. Many people with

excess weight lose up to 2lbs per day without any secondary negative effects. This is because the body is
receiving all the essential dietary elements and does not
suffer from any real deficiencies. But not only is there a
loss of weight, the skin is clearer, there is a regeneration
of the body and there is a feeling of vitality and well-
being.

It also helps to become free from the dependencies of
medicines and stimulants such as coffee, alcohol and
tobacco, and the programme prevents the premature
ageing associated with metabolic illnesses.

5: The full detox programme

Duration

The full detox programme should be carried out for a minimum of five to ten days, but in serious cases and under medical supervision can be prolonged for up to 14 days. (Stanley Burroughs mentions the case of a very overweight person who continued the detox for much longer than that, but we would not advise this unless under strict medical supervision.) During the first three days, the body takes its nourishment from its own reserves, which are stored in the form of gluco-genes (simple sugar) mainly in the blood and the liver, and are easy to absorb. After three days, the body starts to eliminate toxins and to reduce other fatty reserves, which are deposited throughout the body. While this process continues, we don't feel hungry. Only when the deposits are used up does hunger return and the body tells us it is now time to eat again.

The detox programme contains all the vital nutrients that are needed during this time. To carry out the diet once or twice a year has a very positive effect on the health of the body.

A good indicator of the purification progress is the tongue, which sometimes becomes covered with a white coating during the detoxification. When the tongue no longer has its white coating but is clean and pink coloured, the process of purification has finished. (Experiences have shown that in the majority of cases the tongue is still dirty after ten days and sometimes even 14 or 20 days. This indicates that the process of purification has still not finished and that it would be appropriate to repeat the diet on a future occasion.)

During the diet, the body gets rid of the waste and metabolic impurities accumulated over many years through the following body openings (accompanied in some cases by side effects):

- Skin pores
- Intestines
- Urine (darker, sometimes with a strong smell)
- Skin
- Lungs (may produce mucous, bad breath)
- Vagina (may produce an increase in the flow of fluids)
- Mouth (some people experience a bad taste – a drink of peppermint tea helps)

The Detox Drink

Mixing the Natural Tree Syrup & lemon drink is easy. Sometimes it is more convenient to prepare all the mixture for the day in a 2 litre bottle, with the following quantities:

Mixing chart

Batch amount	Syrup	Lemons	cayenne or ginger
300ml water (1 glass)	20ml	Half	small pinch
1800ml (6 glasses)*	120ml	Three	pinch

*Minimum amount per day

Preferably use tepid water but you can also drink it warm or cold.

Cayenne should be added to your personal taste. Some people prefer the drink with a lot of kick while some like it milder. Experiment to find the level that suits you best.

The cayenne pepper dissolves the phlegm and regenerates the blood, which produces more heat in the body. It helps speed the metabolism and also contains many B vitamins, which complement the nutritional value of the Natural Tree Syrup and the lemons. However for those who cannot take cayenne, it can be substituted with ginger.

The Natural Tree Syrup & lemon drink fulfils all the important functions of the cleansing/fasting process:

- It supplies the nutrients necessary for the body's continuing alert functioning, helping to restore the biochemical and mineral balance in tissues and cells and expediting cell regeneration.

- It is quickly and easily assimilated into the bloodstream, freeing the energy of the body used for digestion to other tasks such as detoxification and cell regeneration. The drink supplies very little protein, further aiding the elimination process.

- It provides a liquid medium essential for the efficient flushing of waste from the system.

- The abscorbic acid in the lemons assists the cleansing process, acting as an internal detergent to dissolve excess fats.

Note: Always use fresh lemons or limes, *not* lemonade or concentrated lemon.

Other drinks

During the diet, it is all right to drink a little herbal tea such as peppermint or camomile from time to time.

This helps the purification process and also helps to neutralize the odours of the mouth and body that can appear during the detoxification period.

How much should I drink?

A minimum of six glasses (2 litres) of the mixture should be taken each day. Fluid intake is key to this programme. You are giving your body an internal flush and the Natural Tree Syrup & lemon drink will satisfy your physical hunger and give you energy. Have the mixture ready prepared and as soon as you feel hungry or tired, drink a little of the mixture. Keep drinking it often.

People who are very physically active can increase the dose and make it slightly more concentrated.

Important: Throughout the detoxing programme *no* other foods should be consumed!

As the Natural Tree Syrup & lemon drink contains all the trace elements, vitamins and glucose necessary for ten days, there is no fear once the body has adjusted to the detox, of being hungry.

Use only fresh lemons, if possible organic, the peel of which can be consumed. Never use concentrated lemon juice, frozen lemon juice, or chemically produced lemon drinks.

Natural Tree Syrup, can be obtained from any good health food shop or organic stores, or see page 126. To complete the ten-day diet you will need approximately two litres of syrup.

Programme Length

5-7 Days

The standard version of *The Lemon Detox Diet* is five-seven days. This is the classic version that has been used by thousands of people throughout the world. Many people, when thinking about fasting for the first time, believe they won't be able to make it to seven days but most find that after the second or third day it just gets easier and easier.

7-14 Days

Stanley Burroughs recommended following the programme for ten days because the cleansing gets better the longer the diet continues. By the time you get to the seventh day most people feel so good, that going a few extra days is easy. Going ten-14 days gives the best results by keeping our body in a fasting mode for the fullest length of time.

For more relaxed alternative versions, please see chapter 7.

The eliminatory function is essential

Changing from a solid diet to a liquid one can occasionally produce constipation so it is important to drink plenty of extra water on top of the Natural Tree Syrup & lemon drink.

To aid detoxification, it is useful to help nature with the elimination (bowel movement) process. The body malfunctions when the elimination process is insufficient. For most people it is enough to have a plant infusion laxative. A glass of the infusion should be taken first thing in the morning and last thing at night.

Another good method is to drink a glass of salty water. Mix 1 litre of water with two teaspoonfuls of sea-salt (common kitchen or table salt should *not* be used). The whole litre should be taken in the morning on an empty stomach. In half-an-hour, the salty water cleans the digestive tract very well. This process can be repeated at other times until the bowel is purged. **This method is not recommended for people who have high blood pressure.**

If this water and salt process doesn't work at first, it may be necessary to have a little more or a little less salt, until the appropriate concentration is found. It is good to take a laxative infusion at night, to dissolve waste, and in the morning the salt water to clear the waste. If for any reason you can't or don't want to take the salt water, a laxative infusion may be taken morning and night.

Another very efficient form of cleaning the intestines is by using an enema or undergoing colonic irrigation. This is also an effective way of counteracting the feeling of hunger which can occur on the first day of the diet.

Purging the body is the main point of this detox programme: the impurities that the body is ridding itself of should be evacuated to preclude them being deposited in another part of the body.

No extra foods or pills

Some people want to take vitamin pills or other dietary supplements during the detox programme, but often this is the cause of failure. During the detoxification process the cells get rid of impurities, which accumulate first in the lymphatic glands. Often these get blocked. Only when all impurities are eliminated can the body assimilate correctly again. It is also not recommended to have additional food as this can also endanger the success of the detox programme. The consumption of stimulants such as coffee, alcohol and tobacco also hinder the cleansing process.

The exception to the above is if, for health reasons, you need to take medication that a doctor has prescribed. As a rule, these also obstruct the purification process and are not recommended during the diet, although good results have been obtained during the detox programme with homoeopathic treatments. **However, it is always necessary to consult your doctor regarding the possible effects of stopping any medication.** Consult a doctor who is sympathetic to natural curative methods of this type. (It is not always easy to find such doctors, but it is possible to obtain them from certain associations and natural health magazines.)

Although the success of the detox programme cannot be guaranteed if medication is taken at the same time, experience has shown that even in these cases, cleansing has a beneficial effect on the overall health of the body.

Most people are surprised how well they feel during and after the detox programme. Their energy levels increase substantially, in particular during the second phase of the programme and the majority of people can continue with their normal daily activities without any problems. Many notice that their general state of mind is more positive and their vitality and energy levels increase towards the end.

Another secondary benefit is that people are often able to either stop completely or greatly reduce the intake of analgesics, barbiturates, laxatives and other medications, which they may have been taking on a regular basis before the programme.

Cleansing symptoms

Occasionally during the detox programme, some people suffer from weakness, or even (rarely) need to vomit, and discomfort might occasionally be felt in different parts of the body. This may continue for a day or two and is not a result of any lack of nutrients or vitamins but is simply the effect of the dissolved waste material circulating in the body before final elimination.

Take these symptoms as a positive sign that the detox is working. Before the body's accumulated wastes can be eliminated they first have to be drawn out of the deeper tissues where the body has been storing them.

These symptoms normally disappear after two or three days into the treatment. The diet contains, in liquid form, everything that the body needs for ten or more days. Rest and take things easier if necessary, although the majority of people are able to work as normal. Persevere for the full duration of the treatment; don't give in and don't treat yourself by eating sweets or snacking as this will only compromise the success of the diet.

Headaches
Do not use chemical painkillers. Try to rub a little lavender oil on your temples, close your eyes and relax. If the headache is severe, use a homoeopathic remedy.

Diarrhoea

Do not mistake loose stools for diarrhoea. If you suffer from diarrhoea, drink plenty more water. If the condition lasts for more than 36 hours consult your practitioner.

Insomnia

Brush your body with circular motions. Then soak in a warm bath with a few drops of lavender oil. Try a herbal pillow and drink a cup of lime flower infusion before going to bed. Go to sleep listening to soothing music.

Nausea

Drink some ginger tea.

Bad taste in the mouth

Rinse your mouth and brush your tongue regularly. Drink peppermint tea.

Feeling cold

This is quite normal when you detox. Wrap up well to keep warm.

After the fifth day all the beneficial effects of the treatment will be noticeable.

If the symptoms get worse

If you have any form of chronic illness, for example a skin outbreak, it's possible that the symptoms will become more severe during the treatment. Don't be concerned! This simply means that the body wants to get rid of all the toxins (the skin is an important cleansing organ). As soon as the toxins have left the body, balance is restored and the skin becomes healthier than before.

During this 'cleansing crisis', which occurs during the first day or two, it is possible that no weight is lost, as the incredible intelligence of the body rids itself of that which is most harmful. After this a significant weight loss usually occurs.

Previous problems, or old symptoms can reappear: headaches, nausea, vomiting, halitosis, phlegm, dark urine, secretion of the vagina, diarrhoea, skin eruptions, herpes... don't abandon the treatment: it's the result of the internal cleansing which is working its way out of the system.

Benefits for
alcoholics and smokers

This treatment is excellent for people who want to stop drinking or smoking. The chemical changes and the cleansing which occurs as a result of this treatment are able to reduce or even eliminate the sensation of addiction and multiple symptoms of withdrawal that normally appear. The desire to take artificial stimulants or anti-depressants is reduced, and with time completely disappears. The difficulties, which normally appear when somebody wants to give up smoking, alcohol or other drugs, are greatly reduced by the diet. If you are a heavy smoker, do not stop suddenly, it is better to reduce the daily quantity gradually before you initiate the diet so that you are able to stop smoking by the fourth or fifth day. The body then has time to eliminate the accumulated toxins so that often the physical desire or need to smoke disappears on its own once the treatment is completed. But *The Lemon Detox Diet* can only cure imbalances that originate in the body. If your need to smoke is psychological, you may need to resort to psychological methods or meditation to regain your inner security. However, your feelings of vitality and well-being and the new sensation of a clean inner body will naturally discourage you from smoking.

Exercise

Keep training, but take it easy. Athletes in training may experience a reduction in stamina and are advised to cut back to 60-70% of normal training intensity for the duration of the programme.

Avoid strenuous exercise, because intense exertion may encourage toxins to be reabsorbed rather than eliminated. When we engage in vigorous activity, the body is forced to call upon extra reserves of energy, which it synthesizes from protein and fats. This is a demanding process, distracting the body from its cleansing priorities, and when it is compounded by the release of lactic acid from muscular activity, it only increases the toxic load.

Nevertheless, gentle activities such as yoga or walking are very helpful in waste elimination. The key is finding the right balance between activity and rest. Adequate rest is crucial during the cleanse – while we are resting the body performs vital tasks.

Far from interfering with your training, *The Lemon Detox Diet* is a wise investment for any athlete. Most athletes return to full training after the cleanse with renewed energy and enthusiasm.

Before starting your detox programme, remember the following points.

- Read all the instructions carefully.
- Prepare yourself for the detox and persevere until the necessary changes have taken place.
- Take a cup of laxative tea the night before you start the programme.
- In the morning take a laxative tea or the salt water if you prefer.
- Follow the instructions rigorously.

- After the detox give your body the necessary time to adjust itself to eat again (two-three days).
- Take this wonderful opportunity to break the vicious circle of the bad eating habits!

Typical timetable

Day 1 to 2   Good well-being, perhaps a little hunger. Some people have slight headaches, which last a day or so. Some feel the cold more. This is when the toxins are being drawn out. Be prepared to set aside a little extra time for rest on these days.

Day 3 to 5   Feeling better. Weak or sick patients may find symptoms get worse but this lasts one or two days at the most. With every passing day, most people feel better and better. Feelings of clarity, lightness and well-being grow. Physical cravings for solid food usually decrease dramatically.

Day 6 to 10   Feeling great! It is amazing how good we can feel when we give the body a chance. Most people are rarely hungry and feel healthy and refreshed. Now that most of the toxins are gone, and you've adjusted to the liquid diet you'll probably feel more energetic, clearer, and grounded. You'll have such a feeling of well-being that you'll pity all those poor mortals who have no idea what they are missing.

As blood pressure is reduced during the detox programme, those people with low blood pressure should activate the circulation by means of a short gymnastic exercise routine, some yoga poses, stretching, splashing the whole body with cold water after a hot shower and stimulating the skin with a brush, and drinking a cup of tea.

6: Finishing the programme

Coming back to Earth

It is important that the transition from the liquid diet to regular foods is undergone gradually: the tendency is to eat too much too soon. Since your digestive system has been resting for up to ten days you must give it time to get used to eating normally again.

Plan a gradual transition back to a normal diet, over a two or three day period, introducing more complex foods gradually. From freshly squeezed fruit juices, progress to vegetable juices, raw fruits, raw and steamed vegetables, complex carbohydrates and lastly fats and proteins. Here is a simple model:

Day one

Start the day with a glass of the Natural Tree Syrup & lemon drink, and one orange.
Mid morning: Fresh orange juice.
Lunch: Fruit or vegetable juice.

Tea: Fruit juice or a glass of the Natural Tree Syrup & lemon drink.

Supper: Fresh puréed vegetable soup.

You may also have any herbal teas without caffeine during the day.

Day two

Start the day with a glass of the Natural Tree Syrup & lemon drink, and one orange.

Mid morning: Fresh orange juice.

Lunch: Vegetable soup and fresh fruit.

Tea: Fruit juice or a glass of the Natural Tree Syrup & lemon drink.

Supper: Steamed vegetables, brown rice and salad.

You may also have any herbal teas without caffeine during the day.

Day three

Any breakfast cereal (porridge with Madal Bal Natural Tree Syrup is delicious) with one spoon of Natural Tree Syrup, and one orange.

Mid morning: Fresh orange juice.

Lunch: Roasted vegetables and fresh fruit.

Tea: Fruit juice.

Supper: Vegetable soup, brown rice and fruit salad.

You may also have herbal tea without caffeine during the day.

Do not eat any meat, fish, eggs, bread and sweets. Do not drink soft drinks, tea or coffee during the first three days. From the fourth day you'll be ready to eat 'normally' again.

One of the delightful side effects of *The Lemon Detox Diet* is a heightened awareness of the sensations of taste and smell. By the time you're ready to eat solid food again, your intensified appreciation of the subtleties of taste, texture and fragrance will make this simple experience so much more delectable. Savour the moment.

Extending and repeating the programme

While many people over the years have stayed on the detox programme for many weeks, we never recommend staying on the full detox programme for more than ten days to two weeks. If you are happy with the results, we recommend an interval of roughly as many weeks as you have done days ie: ten weeks for ten days. six weeks for seven days, three weeks for five days and so on.

7. Alternative versions

The relaxed, or Spanish Lemon Diet

Excess weight is probably the most common reason for doing the diet. Many people with excess weight lose up to 2lbs per day, without any secondary negative effects, because the body is receiving all the essential dietary elements and does not suffer from any real deficiencies. But not only is there a loss of weight, the skin is clearer, there is a regeneration of the body and a general feeling of well-being.

The Lemon Detox Diet is versatile and can easily be adapted as a weight management diet and indeed has been adapted to the eating habits of different countries.

The programme was devised in Switzerland as a comprehensive cleansing and detoxification programme. As the programme spread throughout Europe in the 1990s it was adapted to suit different lifestyles and needs. The most popular of these adaptations is known as *The Spanish Lemon Diet*.

Swiss people are serious-minded and thorough and as efficient as the clocks they build. The Spaniards, on the other hand, are renowned for a carefree, relaxed approach to life.

The Spanish Lemon Diet allows the body to purify itself at a slower rate, while still taking in some food. Because of this, to ensure a good purifying effect, the diet should be carried out over a longer period, at least a month and it should be understood that the relaxed version can obviously not achieve the same levels of detoxification as the original programme.

Every night whilst we are asleep we fast, in other words we do not ingest foods and we allow the body to look after itself, to regenerate, purify and recuperate its lost energies – in a large part by the digestion and assimilation of food.

Breakfast breaks this process of recuperation and self-cleaning of the night fast.

The purpose of *The Spanish Lemon Diet* is to prolong this period of night fast, substituting breakfast and/or supper for two or three glasses of Natural Tree Syrup, lemon and water and so offering the body more time to regenerate.

For *The Spanish Lemon Diet* to be effective, it is advisable to remove certain foods which, because of their toxic content, would slow down the cleansing action.

Foods you should avoid

Salt
Red meat
Fried foods
White bread, refined flour and sugar
Lactic products, such as milk, cheeses and yoghurts
Coffee, alcohol and carbonated drinks
Sweets
Processed foods

Food that you can eat

Try to buy organic food. Non-organic is laden with pesticides, the following fruit and vegetables, raw, cooked (slightly) or made into a smoothie.

Fruit: apricots, all berries, kiwi, papaya, peaches, mango, grapes, melons apples, pears, bananas etc.

Vegetables: artichokes, beets, all leafy green vegetables, carrots, cucumber, cauliflower, sweet potatoes, spinach, green and broad beans, peas, bean sprouts, cabbage, kale, etc.

Organic brown rice
Wholemeal bread
Pulses
Steamed fish both white and oily

Chicken without the skin
Nuts and seeds (unsalted)

Teas: Any tea without caffeine, such as peppermint, camomile, dandelion, green tea or mate.

Menu ideas

Breakfast: herbal tea.
From breakfast until lunch: two or three glasses of Natural Tree Syrup & lemon drink.
Lunch: See suggestions below.
From after lunch till evening: two or three glasses of Natural Tree Syrup & lemon drink.

Late evening: laxative drink or tea.

Monday lunch
Avocado and lettuce salad with a dressing of lemon juice and herbs.
Grilled chicken without the skin.
Slice of wholemeal bread with olive oil and garlic (optional).
Fresh fruit.

Tuesday lunch
Light tomato soup.
Baked trout with boiled potatoes and green beans.

Fresh fruit and a handful of nuts.

Wednesday lunch
Baked potato with tuna.
Mixed salad.
Fruit.

Thursday lunch
Pasta with tomato sauce and herbs.
Mixed salad.
Fresh fruit.

Friday lunch
Vegetable soup.
2 slices of brown bread with olive oil and garlic.
Fresh Fruit.

Saturday lunch
Brown pitta bread with ratatouille.
Fresh fruit.
Handful of nuts.

Sunday lunch
Chickpeas with spinach & pine nuts.
2 slices of brown bread with olive oil and garlic.
Fruit salad.

The Spanish Lemon Diet is recommended for those who wish to try *The Lemon Detox Diet* but are unsure about their capacity to last ten days without solid food, and for those who do not feel able or prepared to do the full detox but who need to cleanse their body.

It is also recommended as a preparation for the complete treatment for anyone whose body has high toxicity levels.

Many people continue for one or more weeks with *The Spanish Lemon Diet* after finishing the ten days of the full detox programme. Because the process of detoxification has still not been completed, or they want to lose more weight or simply to counteract a possible desire to eat too much after doing the full *Lemon Detox Diet*.

During the detox, the size of the stomach reduces and it needs and requires less food; after the treatment it is not hunger that makes us eat more than necessary but in many cases the need for sweet foods to celebrate the success of the detox diet and the loss of weight.

The consequences of a lack of moderation in the two weeks following the detox diet can cause quite disagreeable turmoil to the body, such as headaches, cramps, flatulence, fatigue and the return of some of the weight that was lost.

One or two weeks of *The Spanish Lemon Diet* offers an ideal way of avoiding these effects; gently introducing a healthier and balanced food intake and in many cases learning to listen to the innate wisdom of our bodies again: eat when the body tells us to; stop eating when we feel satisfied and not when we are 'full' and, above all, to eat what makes us feel good.

The most important purpose of both the complete detox and the relaxed versions is to make people more conscious of keeping to a healthier general diet, and recognizing their true needs, their eating errors of the past and the effects that food products have on their health and mental and emotional stability.

The 50:50 version

This consists of three days of *The Spanish Lemon Diet,* follow by three days of the full detox programme, followed by another three days of *The Spanish Lemon Diet*. This is an easier way to initiate yourself into the detox if you have never done it before. It also suits some people's social commitments rather better.

The one day a week version

Some people have enjoyed a version of the diet in which they undertake *The Lemon Detox Diet* one day a week, replacing all solid food with the Natural Tree

Syrup & lemon drink on that day. While this does not have the same accumulative effect as the multi-day version of the diet, giving the body a rest one day per week can give the body some chance to catch up on its need to cleanse and detoxify. Going without solid food for a day isn't that difficult and people who have practised this programme have had good long-term weight-normalization results.

8. Tips, trouble-shooting and FAQs

Lack of bowel movement
Remember that chemical drugs, vitamin pills and laxatives should not be taken, use laxative herb teas or salt water (see page 45) and increase your fluid intake.

Insufficient Liquid intake
Countless problems arise because insufficient liquid is taken during the diet. You should drink at least four litres per day (including the diet drink) at least. This ensures that waste material will not be too concentrated in the organs of elimination.

Q: How many calories does the Natural Tree Syrup contain?
A: The energy content of Natural Tree Syrup is 269 kcal per 100 grams.

Q: How many times a year can you repeat the diet?
A: The full detox diet should be carried out twice a year, but it is possible to follow the programme three or

four times a year without detrimental effect. When the programme is followed more frequently, it is recommended that it should not be undertaken for more than ten days.

The Spanish Lemon Diet can be done for one month at a time and repeated every other month.

Q: Will there be an increase in weight immediately after the diet?
A: An increase in weight of one kilo is normal following the treatment, even if your normal diet is correct. But if one eats in moderation, weight will remain stable in the majority of cases. At this time tonic products based on pollen can help a lot, because they supply the body with trace elements and help to maintain the desire to eat within normal limits.

Q:How should one eat after the diet?
A: After the treatment and three days of transition it is recommended that one should gradually change to a wholesome diet. There are many variations of this, but basically denaturalized products and refined products should be avoided, such as white flour and white sugar, preference being given to wholesome organic foods such as cereals, wholemeal flour, salads and raw or steamed vegetables. It is not absolutely necessary to follow a strictly vegetarian diet, but it is always an advantage to reduce the consumption of meat. Don't

risk what you have gained. The most important thing is moderation; use your common sense, the same as in other areas of life. Extremism and fanaticism are out of place.

Q: *Can the diet be carried out while suffering from stomach ulcers?*
A: Originally the *The Lemon Detox Diet* was formulated for the treatment of stomach ulcers. But as these can have different causes, we recommend (as in the case of any medical condition) you carry out the treatment under the supervision of your doctor or experienced health practitioner.

Q: *Can I change the mix of the Natural Tree Syrup & lemon drink?*
A: If you are feeling especially hungry, are being very physically active or have a high metabolism then you may wish to add more syrup to the mix. Try adding the syrup in a 3:2 or 4:2 ratio to the lemon juice. Find a mix that works for you. Some people like more syrup in the mix, some less.

If you cannot have cayenne pepper you may substitute it for ginger.

9. Maintenance advice

Maintaining the achieved weight with the help of pollen supplement

All weight loss can be put back on later through bad diet or poor eating habits, so it is recommended that these be changed. Occasionally a post-dieter might have irrational cravings because of a lack of minerals, which can come about through not eating a wholesome general diet. A pollen supplement provides the body with all the necessary minerals and trace elements. It contributes to maintaining the weight loss achieved through *The Lemon Detox Diet*, suppressing hunger sensations.

Recovery

The cleansing process is followed by the recovery stage: The body must obtain all the nutrients that are needed for it to function well. A wholesome diet is the essential factor to achieve this. If you want to obtain the

maximum benefits from *The Lemon Detox Diet* it is
re... ...lement
fo...

...re

Po... ...nthers
of ...ollen
ha... ...r the
tra... ...analy-
ses ... ...more
than ... ...ntities
not fou... ...nbal-
anced ... ...n our
mo... ...eives
all ...

F... ...n the
nec... ...ood.
The... ...hich
for... ...that
the ... ...are
then ... ...con-
sum...

Pollen helps to maintain an optimum weight

Hunger pangs are often produced when the body lacks certain trace elements. If we eat something that does not contain these nutrients (for example sweet or other refined products) the feelings of hunger soon return. The body needs these nutrients to digest sugars, and if these are lacking in the digestive system, they are taken from areas where they have been deposited, such as the teeth and bones.

The teeth become weak and the lack of trace elements causes a new feeling of hunger. By taking pollen, we are providing the body with almost all of its trace element needs. Hunger diminishes and in this way pollen substantially contributes to maintaining the achieved weight after *The Lemon Detox Diet*.

For how long should pollen be taken?

In my opinion, pollen should be taken for a minimum of two months. Your body, purified by *The Lemon Detox Diet*, needs time to recover and to store all the necessary trace elements. *The Lemon Detox Diet* is always beneficial for the body even if you don't take pollen afterwards. However the pollen complements the diet and can strengthen the body in the long term.

How is pollen consumed?

Pollen is obtained in different ways, but the main factor to be considered is that the tiny grains are covered with a hard shell. This shell is made of one of the most resistant substances existing in nature. In order to obtain the maximum benefit from the multiple active ingredients of pollen it is necessary to open this shell.

Human digestion cannot process more than 10-20% of these pollen granules if the intake is in the form gathered by the bees. The majority of these pollen granules will abandon the body with their valuable contents still intact. In order to obtain any benefit it is necessary to consume relatively large amounts. The normal recommended dosage is between two and three dessertspoonfuls per day.

Up to now the pollen content of capsules and tablets has been produced by crushing these hermetically sealed grains. As the majority of the shells remain intact, these tablets and capsules are practically useless.

Even the bees ferment the pollen before using it as food. In this way, the shells are broken down and the substances within become usable. Normal pollen is relatively easy to harvest using special devices called pollen traps; however, pollen fermented by the bees must be extracted from the panels by hand, and is this is impossible to carry out on a large scale.

The procedure of nitrogenization: (for opening the pollen shells)

Experiments to open the pollen grains have been carried out for some time. Initially they tried to grind the shells but they were so resistant that they remained intact, and the heat generated by this process caused the natural ingredients to be altered and to lose their effect.

A German company has developed a technique that allows almost 100% of the shells to be carefully opened in order to allow the body to process the pollen. Through this technique, the pollen is subjected to extremely low temperatures, until the shells become brittle and can be easily ground. In this way the substances are freed and able to be used despite the low temperature. Afterwards, the pollen is dehydrated and produces the optimum effect even though the quantities are very small.

The Active Apibal capsules, which are produced in this way, have been successfully tested on different age groups. High level sports men and women, athletes, runners and others take Apibal regularly to increase their performance. Other experiments with school children and students showed that the use of Apibal increased their general state of health and improved their concentration and learning ability. Professional people suffering from stress and those of advanced age have also learned how to appreciate the vitalizing effect of pollen. These excellent capsules are recommended whenever the body is exposed to exceptionally difficult circumstances.

10. A survey

Scientific investigations are being carried out on the effects of *The Lemon Detox Diet*, and the following statistics come from a survey of 250 people who followed the programme.

When the programme was followed for ten days, the average weight loss was 5.14kg, with 45% of people losing even more; in other words 23% lost more than 6kg, 15% more than 7kg and 7% more than 8kg. The people were asked how much weight they had lost and the answers were as follows:

Duration of the Detox in Days	Number of People	Los of weight per person (in kg)
1-5	17	2.76
6-9	72	4.36
10	108	5.14
11-20	44	6.27
21-60	9	11.11

Of these 250 people, 108 carried out the detox for the recommended ten days; 89 people did it for a shorter time and 53 for longer.

In 80% of cases, the sensation of hunger disappeared after the first or second day; in the case of those people who had already completed the detox on one or more occasions hunger disappeared more quickly because the body was able to adapt to the diet more easily each time. As soon as there was no intake of food, hunger disappeared. To give up a meal from time to time is no problem for a body that has experienced *The Lemon Detox Diet*.

Intestinal purge also eliminates the sensation of hunger.

Loss of weight in kg	Number of people as a %
2	-
3	10%
4	20%
5	25%
6	23%
7	15%
8	7%

It should be kept in mind that 18% did not follow the instructions to the letter and during the detox diet had, among other things solid food: so, if the rules had been followed, the average weight loss would have been even greater!

Longer & shorter diets

More than 20% of people carried out the detox diet for more than ten days, in one extreme case for 61 days. The lady who persevered for 61 days was very positive, which demonstrates the inoffensive character of this treatment, even for a long period of time. **We would, however, recommend medical supervision if anyone wishes to follow the diet for more than two weeks or suffers from a medical condition.**

Those people who carried out the diet for less than six days also experienced positive results, but a lasting effect can only be found after six-seven days. In the group that carried out the diet for six-nine days, the weight loss was only slightly below that of the ten-day group.

90% were enthusiastic

174 people gave the diet the best evaluation possible with 'very good', 49 people considered it 'good'. These figures show that 88% were totally satisfied – a result that not many diets obtain.

The absolute majority want to follow it again, among other things for the feeling of well-being experienced during the treatment.

What do you think about the diet?

Very Good	69.6%
Good	19.6%
Average	4.0%
Poor	2.0%
No opinion	2.4%

More than 80% of people were happy not only with the loss of weight but with other positive changes. Many said that their skin improved, their energy levels increased and they achieved a more positive state of mind. They also mentioned improvements in their hair condition; sleep patterns, better circulation, the condition of the nails and the diminishment of chronic pains. Many felt sorry that the detox programme was not better known and many wished to repeat it on a future occasion.

Problems with the detox

Approximately half the number of people did not have any problems and the majority of the others encountered only minor difficulties that are directly related to the internal cleansing of the body: 15% mentioned mild headaches at the beginning, 12% mild or temporary tiredness, approximately 11% mild weakness and approximately 6% hunger or the desire to eat sweets. Other problems appeared only in individual cases and were limited mainly to pains in different parts of the body – reduction in clarity of vision during the first few days: and a feeling of coldness as no foods are being burned.

Overall results

The majority of those who carried out the detox programme supported it completely. More than 80% of the people noticed positive changes during and after the diet. As well as the loss of weight, they mentioned above all a greater state of well-being, which can be considered a result of the internal cleansing that was carried out during the detox programme.

11. Spiritual cleansing

Up to now we have looked at the *The Lemon Detox Diet* almost exclusively from the point of view of cleansing the body. But this detox programme also has a purifying effect over the mental state and a positive effect on general well-being.

The Romans used the expression: *mens sana in corpore sano* – a healthy mind in a healthy body. Another well-known proverb says that man is what he eats. As far as macrobiotics are concerned, diet is a decisive factor in a person's character. A Japanese naturopath asked once if people in the West were cold and aggressive because they ate so much meat. It is increasingly obvious that food has something to do with conscience.

From time immemorial, holy men and monks have carried out periods of fasting to purify the mind, the emotions and the spirit. The list of great thinkers and philosophers who practised and recommended fasting is impressive: Christ, Mohammed, Buddha, Moses, Elijah, Hippocrates, Galen, Paracelsus, Pythagoras,

Socrates, Plato, Aristotle, St Francis and Mahatma Gandhi:

I fast for greater and physical and mental efficiency.
Plato

Prayer takes us halfway towards God, fasting takes us to the gates of Heaven. **Mohammed**

As my body loses its superfluous weight, my being becomes more luminous and my spiritual being clearer and more resolute. **Buddha**

Jesus also talked about fasting and put it into practice during the forty days and nights that he spent in the desert.

The Lemon Detox Diet provides an excellent opportunity to purify not only the body but also the mind. Many letters provide evidence that the cleansing effect of the *The Lemon Detox Diet* greatly increases the capacity to concentrate: this does more than just compensate for any possible minor physical weakness, particularly in people who carry out some form of intellectual work.

At the same time it is noticed that the mind becomes more receptive and positive. The diet activates the right hemisphere of our brain for creativity, intuition and perception. Other effects are those of tranquillity and lightness of spirit. Many people say they feel like new. Many who have up to now been too materialistic find that they become much more aware of their inner being.

Losing excess weight, detoxifying the body and re-establishing a healthy balance are obviously very important results of the detox programme. But for many people, the psychological effects are almost more important. We should not underestimate the value of achieving new eating habits as a consequence of the detox diet, because since the beginning of time and throughout the world, this step also signifies the beginning of a new life in which man places more value on his inner self than in the eating pleasures.

For many, the importance of these values is increasing day by day. More and more people are rejecting pre-conceived ideas that external values are all important and, as a result, look for ways and means of exploring their inner world. The art of meditation is of great value in achieving this. Although the majority of techniques used nowadays come from the East, these methods can be practised and can be of great use to Western man. Meditation techniques bring together this ancient art with all the requirements of life in modern Western society. With their help, many people have reached the conclusion that happiness in life and deep satisfaction are not only desirable but can actually be obtained by turning their back on the world. One of the main objectives of meditation is the internal balance and the spiritual purification of man. *Purity on its own is able to resolve 99% of human problems,* says spiritual leader Sri Chinmoy. Profound experiences become possible only when the human being has been purified.

In that way interior purification is of prime importance for a deeper and more satisfying life. While meditation constitutes a direct way towards spiritual purification, a programme such as *The Lemon Detox Diet* begins with purification of the body. One complements the other and often one leads to the other. As you can see this diet can give you more than you expected!

Many people find that one of the greatest benefits of *The Lemon Detox Diet* is that they gain a deeper perspective about themselves. During the cleanse, going without food is not the hardest part. It is overcoming the emotional and mental attachments to food that is difficult. Most of us aren't even aware of these attachments. We become more empowered when we are freed from them. We gain a deeper understanding of ourselves and a stronger ability to control our desires and attachments instead of them controlling us. This is very spiritually uplifting as we become more aware of ourselves, who we are and what we are capable of.

The Lemon Detox Diet can be a means of spiritual

renewal and self-discovery. For those interested in exploring this facet of cleansing we recommend meditation as a pathway to deeper awareness.

A simple exercise

As the body is cleansed and purified, so it seems our thoughts become clearer, our minds less confused and distracted. Many feel a sense of new life, free of worries, fears and anxieties. Here is a simple concentration/meditation exercise to practise in conjunction with *The Lemon Detox Diet*.

Set aside ten minutes per day; preferably early in the morning before you enter into your daily routine.

Choose a place where you can sit alone peacefully, perhaps a corner of your room which is kept clean. It is helpful to set up a small sacred space, a place with flowers and a candle or a crystal. Play some peaceful meditative music and light some incense. Alternatively select a peaceful spot outside amidst nature.

Sit comfortably either in a chair or on a cushion with your spine erect to keep you alert. Try to focus your attention on your breath, focusing on each inhalation and exhalation. As you inhale you feel that you are breathing in a feeling of peace and calm and as you exhale feel that you are releasing any feelings of tension or anxiety and that you are allowing the peaceful feeling to spread throughout your body. Finally, try to allow your breath to become very calm and quiet, imagining that if someone placed a feather in front of your nose, it would hardly move.

To focus your mind, breathe in as you slowly count to five, hold for two counts and then exhale again for five counts. This must be comfortable without straining your lungs. Try to make the counting absolutely regular, rhythmical. Feel that nothing else exists in the world apart from your breathing and counting. This is the only task that matters. If other distracting thoughts enter your mind try to let them go and return your focus to your breath.

After a few minutes of counting, feel that what you are breathing is not air but solid peace. Imagine that this peace enters directly into the depths of your heart. From there it flows outwards, permeating your heart, mind, emotions and whole physical body.

In the same way, you can breathe in any quality you need: patience, love, power, tolerance and joy. During the course of *The Lemon Detox Diet,* breathe in the feeling of purity. Feel this purity flowing from the centre of your chest, through your body, through your mind and your emotions. Consciously imagine you are breathing out all the toxins and waste from your system and that they are being replaced with vibrant energy, enthusiasm and joy.

When finishing your meditation practice, gradually return your awareness to your surroundings.

Simple daily exercise is also a great part of the spiritual side of cleansing. Cardiovascular exercise can be like a meditation when we try to keep our mind focused on our breath or in the experience of the exercise. Try not to allow your thoughts to focus on the past or the future. Try to keep it still and focused on the exercise and your breath or, if you are outside, the beauty of the surrounding nature.

12. The Lemon Detox Diet offers more

Up to now we have considered *The Lemon Detox Diet* from the aspect of reduction and purification of the whole body. But for its creator Stanley Burroughs it was first and foremost part of a natural curative method – which is more far-reaching. Before going into details we would like, for clarity's sake, to look for a moment at the ideas of this man on the success or otherwise of traditional medicine and the origin of illnesses.

In the opinion of Stanley Burroughs: *All curative systems are limited in their degree of effectiveness*. This comes from the lack of global understanding of the independent functions of the body, which often hide the real cause of the illness.

There are a lot of factors that influence the healing of the body. Physical exercise, sport, physical work and also Hatha Yoga, keep the body in good condition and are particularly recommended during the detox programme. Above all, in these times of inertia a conscious training routine of this type is important.

Often a good masseur can be a positive contributor, massaging those parts of the body that are painful or tense. A massage relaxes, helps the circulation, breaks up blood clots and stimulates the organs and cells of the body. This system is an ancient healing method and is extremely successful. Steam baths are also beneficial, if they are carried out in conjunction with massage and physical exercise. Another form of treatment is the use of medicinal plants which supply the body with those elements that are lacking and can make up for deficiencies that result from an incomplete diet.

All these types of alternative medicine are complementary to *The Lemon Detox Diet* and often increase its effect.

The origin of chemical medication

In recent times, science has started to isolate various components of medicinal plants, to make them more effective. During this process, many balancing elements are lost from the plants and secondary effects occur. With the advancement of modern chemistry, drugs have become stronger and undesirable secondary effects are now more dangerous.

When drugs do not produce the desired effect, psychology is added to the treatment to overcome the limitations. New practices are constantly included, often in opposition to traditional medicine, but even today many illnesses are still incurable.

At other times doctors resort to surgical operations in an attempt to achieve what has not been possible through medication. Success is doubtful especially in the case of chronic illnesses. Even though many millions of pounds have been invested, science has not advanced much in this region. In modern times the number of health practitioners who are returning to the simple rules of nature is increasing, and in this way new natural methods are developed, which in some ways are better than traditional medicine.

The necessity of global understanding

Systems lacking in the global understanding of man – both physical and spiritual – are condemned to failure. The limitation will last the same time as partial understanding. Negative secondary effects and failures will stop only when we apply the perfect laws of nature. Only when there is a complete assurance that a medicine really works, can it be called true and correct.

As soon as man understands and applies the laws of natural health and its curative effects, complications and illnesses usually disappear. The types of illnesses can be distinguished, like the leaves of a tree; but they are all leaves from the same tree. We do not need to know all the laws of treatment and perfect health; all we need to know is how to apply these laws and our creator will do the rest.

The simplicity, integrity and efficiency of natural methods of treatment, which are spreading little by little, are fascinating. Often it is difficult for somebody through normal understanding to recognize that these methods really work. Whether one understands it or not, the most important thing is that it is as it is.

Although knowledge of curing with the help of nature seems new and revolutionary, in reality it has existed for thousands of years – all it needs is for competent people to bring it to light again. It is not a question of trying to bring something new into the world, but to bring something ancient to light, something that has existed forever, and to allow these simple laws to act in our favour. It would seem that the principles of *The Lemon Detox Diet* are contrary to everything we have believed and learned. But this does not stop them being effective and true. Before trying to deny these facts, you can try out the diet for yourself, to discover from personal experience whether or not it works.

Stanley Burroughs always concluded that the body would cure itself, because according to him, *the capacity of the human body to cure itself is unlimited*. We only need to give the body the opportunity to do so; *The Lemon Detox Diet* together with other natural treatments makes this possible.

13. Epidemics & viruses

Where do epidemics come from?

Stanley Burroughs wondered where epidemics came from. His explanation was very revealing.

From time immemorial, epidemics have occurred. The reason for this is still not well known. In years gone by it was believed to be an act of the devil or a punishment from the gods. Today it is believed that they are contagious diseases spread by pathogenic agents. This belief has become a monster in the field of medicine.

New drugs, poisons and antibiotics have always been found to destroy what has been considered the cause of the illness. But despite many investigations being carried out, humanity continues to suffer from these infirmities.

Illness, ageing and premature death, according to Stanley Burroughs, are the result of accumulated toxins, blood clots in different parts of the body and as a consequence a weakened immunological system.

These toxins crystallize and are deposited in the joints, muscles and in the innumerable cells of the body.

Orthodox medicine presumes our body is healthy until pathogenic agents or viruses come to attack it. But in reality the material that makes up our cells and organs is not healthy and it is because of this that illnesses and disease can attack. There are specific areas of the body where unusable waste products are deposited. Often they appear in the lymphatic glands, or in the liver, pancreas, stomach, intestines and the heart, hindering the healthy function of these organs.

These tumours appear in the form of fungi. Their growth and propagation depend on the quantity of unusable wastes that are in the body. If the deterioration continues, the tumours grow and begin to control the situation. The fungi absorb the toxins and try to eliminate the waste from the organs. This forms part of a natural plan to free the body of illness. When we stop feeding these fungi and start to cleanse out the system, we stop their growth and propagation; the body dissolves them and gets rid of them, because they cannot live on healthy tissue. There is a simple theory of law that can explain this: *nature does not produce anything it does not need and never keeps what it cannot use.* All the unusable material and waste are dissolved by bacteria into a new usable form or eliminated from the body. All those cells, which are weak and deficient because of a bad diet, are also broken down and eliminated.

We spend a great part of our lives creating illnesses and the rest of the time we spend eliminating them and dying in the process. A bad understanding of these truths leads civilized nations to look for a magic cure through spells, witchcraft and in innumerable poisons and repulsive drugs. Generally these are worse than useless, because in no way can they eliminate the cause of the illnesses. They can only add misery to suffering and shorten life even more. Various articles in magazines and books show that many new illnesses and disorders actually develop through orthodox methods and clinics. The more we look for miraculous new medicines, the more we get involved in the complex diversity of types of illness. But as always, comprehension and the simple answer have been the best way to eliminate illness. If we learn how to eat the correct foods and avoid those that are toxic, we will be able to detoxify our system, build a healthy body and free ourselves at last from a large number of illnesses.

I hope this short resumé of the theories of Stanley Burroughs gives you an insight into the ideas of the famous naturopath and an understanding of the principles behind *The Lemon Detox Diet*.

14. Comments by practitioners

I have tested it myself and am now introducing it in practice. I can vouch that it tastes good, is easy to sustain over 5-10 days, gives a rapid detox, and is suitable for a wide variety of patients.

Dr Janine Leach BSc PhD ND DO Hon MFPHM

Speciality: Naturopath

The main objective of our preconceptional programme is to renew the adipose tissues of the body, in order to reduce the amount of all sorts of fat soluble synthetic chemicals such as PCBs and dioxins. During a weekend, there is no food available other than a specially designed cocktail made from Natural Tree Syrup (a mixture of maple syrup, and palm tree syrup) and lemon juice. Cayenne pepper is added after dilution (a way to slightly increase the body temperature). The cocktail can be consumed at any time without any restriction. Its mineral content is exceptionally rich. The ratio of zinc to manganese to iron is ideal (in the region of 5:2:1). The ratio of calcium to magnesium is around 2.5:1 and the ratio of potassium to sodium around 10:1. The lemon juice represents the main source of natural vitamin C.

Dr Michel Odent, Primal Health Research Center

Speciality: Obstetrician

Even using the Madal Bal Natural Tree Syrup as a meal replacement once a day can support a healthy and steady weight loss regime. At the same time, one gains consistent energy levels to face life's demands. This works well combined with homoeopathy for full optimization of one's health.

Dr Elizabeth Adalian R S Hom

Speciality: Homoeopathy teacher and clinician

One thing that really impresses me about The Lemon Detox Diet *is that energy levels remain high, so you can continue with normal leisure and work activities.*

Mr Ian Barret BSc ND DO MRN MAO

Speciality: Naturopath, Holistic Health Consultant

I find The Lemon Detox Diet *very useful for women wanting to conceive – many people change their diet when they are actually pregnant. So much better to be prepared for pregnancy.*

Ms Emma Cannon

Speciality: Pre-natal care, pregnancy, women's health advisor, acupuncturist

Very useful to kick-start dietary changes that can be permanently incorporated in a patient's lifestyle. Good way of eliminating toxins and habits, makes healing easier, giving energy to the liver where adrenal toxins are commonly found.

Mr Trevor Gunn BSc (Hons) LCH RS Hom
Speciality: Homoeopath

One of the best detox diets around. The results are excellent and long lasting. I have now started to incorporate The Lemon Detox Diet *into my clinic.*

Ms Marcia Harewood ND MRN DO MH DNI
Speciality: Osteopath, Naturopath, Herbal Medicine practitioner, Iridologist

After testing the tasty Natural Tree Syrup myself, I felt great, dropped a dress size and have more energy. Now I am introducing it as part of my detox workshops and am recommending it to clients.

Debbie Fraser, BSc BWY dip PGCE
Speciality: Yoga teacher, Yoga therapist, Detox workshops therapist, Reiki practitioner, Thermal Auricular therapist, Indian head masseuse

Wonderful and energizing.

Mr Paul Lefever
Speciality: Complementary Therapy adviser plus teaching insight meditation teacher

I used The Lemon Detox Diet firstly for myself and was so pleased with the results that I now recommend it to my clients. It achieves profound results physically, emotionally and spiritually and the body deeply cleanses itself of accumulated toxins.

Ms Carol Melling

Speciality: Reiki Master and teacher, Kundalini Yoga teacher, Healing Sound therapist

Excellent to use for detox and fasting, especially helpful where people have busy lifestyles and have little time for juice fasting. Also very helpful in retraining eating patterns to combat overeating.

Ms Jayne Kirtley MRN RN (ND, Registered Nurse)

Speciality: Naturopathy

Can't recommend it highly enough. I use it to fast/detox before giving Reiki attainments. Best hot!

Rev Barbara M. Occleshaw

Speciality: Craniosacral balancing, Reiki Master, Yoga teacher

The Lemon Detox Diet is the ideal spring-clean because you can adapt it to your own needs. It is surprisingly refreshing and you don't feel deprived at all! I thoroughly recommend it once or twice a year.

Mrs Martina Watts BA (Hons) Dip ION

Speciality: Clinical Nutritionist, Adults and children with digestive immune disorders

The Lemon Detox Diet *is the only fast that we recommend as part of our detox program. It is excellent.*
Mr Donatus Roobeek
Speciality: Holistic practitioner

I recommend The Lemon Detox Diet *to clients as a highly effective, adaptable and safe method of fasting.*
Mrs Penny Scrivener BANT ECNP
Speciality: Nutritional Therapy, Bicom Bioresonance, and scenar

I found this product excellent for myself and have recommended it to patients who I thought would benefit from it ... very 'do-able' and extremely beneficial.
Ms Grania Stewart-Smith DO
Speciality: Osteopath, Bioresonance practitioner

A safe, natural and effective way to detox and control weight. Great for busy working lives.
Mrs Allison Walker MIIR (Regd) MAR ART (Regd)
The Marjorie Centre for Complementary Health
Speciality: Reflexology with holistic health advice

Personally I have used the syrup for the detox diet several times and recommend it to my patients.
Dr Jeffrey Mc Tavish
Speciality: Chiropractor

I was amazed at the effectiveness of the diet and its simplicity makes it easy to follow when travelling away from home. I found the drink was very satisfying, I didn't feel hungry or weak at all and was able to carry on with work and activities as usual. I have recommended it to many colleagues and patients.

Mrs Jill Carter

Speciality: Nutritionist

I enjoyed doing The Lemon Detox Diet *and felt satisfied – not hungry at all (surprisingly!). Sight detox symptoms on third evening. Lost 6lbs. Will be actively recommending it to colleagues and clients.*

Ms Jayne Walker

Speciality: Aromatherapy, Kinesiology, Bowen technique, Allergy/food intolerance, Detoxification

A comfortable way of detoxifying.

Dr Tom Greenfield, Spring Gardens Clinic

Speciality: Blood group diet, Fasting, Cranial Osteopathic treatment

15. International referrals

I am a professional sportsman and a Tae-kwondo coach. I use the Natural Tree Syrup & lemon drink while I take part in competitions as it provides all the necessary nutrients and at the same time is easily digested. It has the added advantage of helping to control my weight.

Javier Sanchez, Tae-kwondo coach – El Prat Barcelona, Spain

I came across your book about The Lemon Detox Diet *a year-and-a-half ago. I am delighted with this detox programme, which I repeat every six months. I have recommended it to several friends and they are also delighted with the results.*

E H – Zurich, Switzerland

Thank you! My rheumatic headaches have disappeared after I did The Lemon Detox Diet. *It is fantastic!*

Mrs A C (40 years) – Marseille, France

For many years I tried to lose 15lbs without result. With The Lemon Detox Diet I have lost 17lbs. In the first four days I lost 4lbs, in the following four days I lost another 8lbs. I am now 2lbs below the 15lbs that I originally wanted to lose.

I did not have any problem during the diet. I don't feel hungry or thirsty and I walk with my wife over 7km every day. I am delighted. I was very sceptical about the programme but I now recommend it to everybody.

Mr E V (45 years) – Munich, Germany

I lost 5kg with your diet two months ago and I have not regained any weight. I am thrilled!

J K (56 years) – Verona, Italy

Before the diet I had 4.2 cholesterol. Now, after ten days on the diet my cholesterol reading is 1.7. I have also lost 7kg (14lb).

Enrique B – Barcelona, Spain

I am a pensioner and rather fat. I did The Lemon Detox Diet for ten days drinking eight glasses of the mixture per day. I lost 10kg in ten days! For me this is an incredible success and I will recommend it to all my friends. Many thanks.

Mr S B (67 years) – Barcelona, Spain

16. Comments from UK users

I just wanted to write and let you know that The Lemon Detox Diet *was superb! The Natural Tree Syrup was surprisingly enjoyable to drink and completely curbed my food cravings I felt better than ever after a little bit and at least three people a day commented on how healthy and glowing I looked I will be integrating the detox programme into my lifestyle on a regular basis.*

J H – London E14

I have lost 9lbs in six days. I can't tell you how grateful I am for your guidance and courtesy. The product is wonderful! I felt bad (giddy and hungry) until the fourth day but now I sleep better, with no more headaches, depressions or sciatica. and I have slightly more energy and more will-power. I feel happy and floating on air. I just can't imagine what I shall be like on the eighth day. Look out world – here I come.

Ms S – London

Not easy, but very rewarding. There is the weight loss which is extremely welcome but that's not the main point. It's self-discipline, and the realization of how little food is actually needed; it's the knowledge that the body is being given the best possible assistance in its natural cleansing process. And at the end of it all, real appreciation of healthy food again.
Mr P H

I've done ten days and enjoyed it enormously. I felt very good when I had finished – and no food cravings. It really was not very difficult … From now on I can use the syrup when I am on the move (it was difficult to carry all my special foods with me before). Knowing that I can live happily on so little solid food is very liberating!
Ms C – Dumfriesshire

My mum and I each did a five day detox and found the experience made us feel wonderful even though the first three days were hell! … We are hoping to do a detox every three or four months just because we feel so fit and healthy, inside and out. My mum and I both practise yoga and exercise regularly and I found that we had much more enthusiasm towards working out and felt much more gain.
Miss W – Teeside

I'd never done a detox regime before. I was attracted by the simplicity of The Lemon Detox Diet *and the beauty of the syrup tin. I was surprised and delighted to discover that the lemon and syrup mixture tasted delicious and further more assuaged all hunger, which made the programme easy to sustain. I had thought of adopting a 'Spanish' rather than 'Swiss' approach, as I needed to eat with some people during my detox period. I found that eating at lunchtime 'Spanish' style was very uncomfortable, very badly tolerated, whereas a light meal on the occasional evening presented no problems.*

Ms K – London

Whilst on the diet I felt slim, healthy and no longer a food slave.

Ms J – Huddersfield

I completed the ten day programme even though I only intended to do five days as it was my first time. Even now, I am amazed to say how easy I found the whole experience. I never really felt hungry at all, but some days I just fancied a change of diet. It was never an awful struggle. I did experience headaches, tiredness and a bad taste in my mouth for the first four days. From the fifth day I felt really wonderful! I was walking regularly with the dog daily and I remember attempting a very steep hill, which I usually avoid because it is such a very exhausting climb. That day I could have run up it! I have never had so much energy. My skin felt so soft and clear and several dry patches had gone. I had lost 12lbs by the end of the course. I am changing my diet for the better and have not touched caffeine or alcohol since.

Ms P – Surrey

I have had a weight problem for about 15 years, and I have tried every diet imaginable, including diet tablets, drinks and patches ... all of which didn't work at all for me, so to say that I was a little apprehensive at first would be an understatement! I started my programme on a Wednesday, so first thing in the morning I weighed myself in at 11 stone. I opted for the ten-day plan, and started to take my drinks at regular intervals, but all I could manage was five cups on the first day. I felt a bit light-headed on day two, and had a slight headache. No one could have prepared me for my findings when I got on the scale in the morning of day two, I had lost 5lbs, on day three I was well into it, because the massive reductions gave me the incentive I needed to carry on. By day four I was feeling on top of the world, but passing a lot of mucus. I managed to get some laxative tea and took some on day four, and I was quite astounded by what I had passed when the tea took effect. By day ten I weighed myself, I was 10 stone; I have lived through

Christmas and New Year and not gained an ounce back. I wanted to thank you for finding this miracle for people like me.

Mrs P A – Leicester

I was very impressed with how I felt after the diet. I originally tried to fast completely, but having a very active job, I found that after the first day I felt unwell, so switched to eating lunch and replacing the other meals with the Natural Tree Syrup & lemon drink. I will definitely do it again and I think I'd like to try it for longer next time.

Ms L – email

After experiencing the lemon detox for five days I now have a feeling of well-being and have adopted sensible eating habits. I look forward to doing the programme soon for ten days.

M M – Co Dublin

I recently completed the ten-day lemon detox. The system was easy to use and the diluted Natural Tree Syrup & lemon drink was very pleasant. I can recommend this system to anyone. I thoroughly enjoyed it. I didn't experience any side effects at all and felt well throughout. My energy levels were just as high, even though I had no food at all for the duration. It is important to follow the instructions carefully, in par-

ticular to be vigilant in preventing constipation. This could be the reason I escaped the toxic reactions. I practise and teach yoga every day, and because yoga is an internal cleanser, build up of toxins and poisons are prevented. so I didn't lose much weight, maybe 2-3lbs, but this was not my motivation anyway, as I am not overweight. I intend to repeat this detox programme every six months.

Ms S – Nelson, Lancs

I completed the five day fast successfully, although it was a great challenge! I mostly felt well during it, but if I'm honest I was hungry! However, I felt and do still feel well, I have more energy, and a new relationship with food. Weight loss was a welcome bonus and I continue to look and feel better. I shall do the fast again – though I think it will always be five days rather than ten for me.

PT – Kent

I am going to do the five day detox again but I want to get the larger tin because I am always inviting people to try it. I really enjoyed the diet, and suffered none of the side effects that you said could occur. My skin was great, my energy levels were high (I did Astanga yoga during the diet, as well as run around with my two young boys) and I only rarely felt hungry. I did lose 12lbs in weight, which I was *delighted about and which has stayed off even after Christmas. When my five days came to an end I thought I would LOVE to eat again, but if I had any syrup left I would have still wanted to drink that for the first morning. I really missed my drink and tried to mix teas and lemon to see if I could find a substitute. Without success!*

B B – London

I just thought I should let you know the amazing result of my detox programme. First of all I am very energetic, I did the whole ten days and am able now to climb to the third floor to work every morning without gasping for breath. My constant craving for coffee is under control; I now only drink one cup of coffee a day only for the love of it and not to keep alert … I am satisfied with water. I have lost 5kg and it is two weeks now and I still haven't put it back on. I am so happy about this. In the past, when I've fasted I had always put the weight back on within a short period. I am feeling so good I think I will do another five days after a couple of months.

Ms A – email

Just to let you know I've had another 'session' with the Madal Bal lemon detox and it has gone very well – yet again! I have lost weight – about 10lbs – so now I am about the right weight, which is very nice. What

is even more exciting is that my toe has got complete-
ly better. I damaged it as a schoolgirl as a result of
ballet dancing and it became arthritically inflamed.
Since I did the lemon detox it has returned to normal.
I can't tell you how fantastic that is. Let's hope it
stays that way!
N H – London SE22

I did The Lemon Detox Diet *for ten days and lost*
12lbs in weight. I felt great after the detox. Also a
lump on my neck (which had puzzled several doctors
in London) disappeared!
S – Kent

The Lemon Detox Diet *was a great success for the*
following reasons – my skin feels a lot better; my hair
is shining again; I feel that I'm back in control of my
eating habits; and I lost 12lbs. I know some of this
will go back on, but it's a great incentive to eat sensi-
bly.
Ms P – Leeds

I undertook the detox for five days, as it was my first
time. I did enjoy the Natural Tree Syrup & lemon
drink and despite having to drink a lot of it, I did not
get bored or sick of the taste. Over days three and
four, I felt tired and a bit lacking in energy, but
managed to persevere. By day five, I really felt great

and had a burst of energy and positive feelings. I also noticed problem patches of skin improved and many people commented on how well and 'sparkly' I looked. Ordinarily I am quite pale and can look run down, but my family have all noticed how healthy I have looked since completing the detox. On commencing eating normally once again, I was pleasantly surprised that I did not have great urges to overeat, but was quite happy to eat small amounts of very simple food. Since returning to a normal diet I have noticed a great lack of desire for processed and artificial foods and tastes and a continued preference for natural and plain options. On the whole, the experience of the detox was a most positive one and I definitely noticed and felt the benefits.

Mrs S – Aberdeenshire

I was amazed to find that, at the end of eight days, I had lost 12lbs of excess weight. I also feel more energetic and well rested than I have for many years. I found the programme easy to stick to and convenient to follow, and will be recommending it to friends, colleagues and clients... Thank you to you and your organization for providing this excellent and enjoyable way of achieving and maintaining excellent health in body and mind.

Mrs C – Lanarkshire

It is now ten days since I completed the diet and I feel absolutely fantastic. I have got so much energy. Food has taken on a different meaning and taste altogether and although it was quite a challenge (which I love anyway) I would definitely do it again. I imagine the first time is definitely the hardest – but now I know about the various stages ie, I can take homoeopathic headache pills and salt for the cramps. So I shall be better prepared for next time. I have kept up good habits and I find myself wanting to eat healthily – but enjoying it at the same time. I have recommended it to my friends and family, because I really think there is so much to be gained from the diet. In short, I felt I rose to the challenge and reaped so many rewards.
Ms S – email

I have been on the lemon detox for four days now and feel wonderful with a 4lb weight loss so far. I'm doing the relaxed version, as my willpower won't stretch to the full-blown programme. I feel so cleansed.
Ms A – email

I could not believe how quickly the detox kicked in. I started on Monday at 8am and when I sat down at 4.30pm, I could not keep my eyes open and my head was muggy. I could not stay out of my bed. I was in bed from 6.45pm to 9.30am the next day. Slight tiredness and my head feeling as though it was filled with

*cotton wool for the next four days. It was very easy,
no hunger, but I found it difficult to build up the
drink to six a day. Drinking water was no problem as
I drink a lot of it anyway. Elimination was a slight
problem, but toxins certainly escaped through pores.
It is now three days since I completed the programme
and I feel very good. Keeping to a light diet has
helped me set a healthy diet, cutting out coffee, in
between nibbles, and being more aware of balancing
my diet. My head is now very clear, and my energy
levels are raised. I think I was too ambitious, but I
will return to the detox probably about Easter time –
easing into it on the Spanish system.*

R – Burnt Island

*I have now completed my first fortnight with the
syrup and lemon drink and have to say that I feel
better inside than I have done for years! I did the
extended version purely because there were things in
the house that needed using, mainly vegetables, so I'm
full to the brim with soup of one sort or another.*

Ms D – email

This is now my fifth day on The Lemon Detox Diet
*and I am feeling pretty good. I have lost approximate-
ly 7lbs. It has not been too bad considering I have
never done a full detox before, the only day that was
bad was the second day, when I suffered from a severe*

*headache, but survived that. It's surprising how I
don't feel hungry but as you said it is a mental challenge. I am really enjoying the diet and would
recommend it to anyone. I probably won't do it for
any longer than seven days and might start to introduce fruit juices and fruit as of tomorrow, as I really
don't want to lose any more weight.*
Ms A M – Carfin

*What a wonderful treatment. I could have stayed on
the detox for much longer. I feel so much better for it.*
Ms C – Bucks

*My detox went well. I did require will-power, but not
as much as I thought though. I still cooked for the
family every evening (keeping the lemon drink
nearby). It has helped change my attitude to food,
realizing how much we eat out of habit and boredom.
We had friends over for dinner, they cooked and ate,
and I enjoyed their company. Although during the
first four days of the plan I had muscle cramps, but
once they had passed, my legs felt lighter and more
flexible. I seem to have lost my taste for tea, coffee
and dairy products.*
Ms L – Cornwall

17. And that's not all …

Other Uses

If you have any left over, the Natural Tree Syrup is an excellent sweetener. It makes a perfect alternative to refined sugar or artificial sweeteners, because the quality of its natural sugar is much superior to that of refined sugar – it also contains much less calories.

The Natural Tree Syrup is particularly tasty with:

Breakfast cereals
Yoghurt
Pancakes
Fruit salad
Ice cream
In fruit smoothies

Recipes

Sent to us by Natural Tree Syrup users

Tofu oriental with Natural Tree Syrup and curry sauce

1 tbsp oil; 1 onion; 500g Tofu, cut into small cubes;
1 small apple; 1 banana; 1 tsp sea salt; 1 clove
garlic, crushed; 3-4 tsp curry sauce; 2-3 tsp soy
sauce; 2 tsp Natural Tree Syrup; handful of currants
and some chopped almonds. 100ml cream and a little
water.

Fry the onion and Tofu. Slice the apple and the
banana and add to the pan. Add the other ingredients
and stir. Serve this delicious sauce with rice.

Natural Tree Syrup & Banana cream

3 ripe bananas; juice and grated rind of half lemon;
3 tbsp Natural Tree Syrup; 2 plain yoghurts; 150g
cottage cheese or Tofu; cream.

Beat everything together and serve with the Filled
Pancakes.

Filled Pancakes

3 eggs; 3 tbsp flour; pinch of salt; 300ml milk;
1 tbsp butter; 1-2 tbsp Natural Tree Syrup.

Beat all the ingredients together and leave to rest for one hour. Use the batter to make very thin pancakes and serve.

For the stuffing:
2 tsp orange juice; 1-2 tbsp sultanas; 150g cheese or Tofu; 2 tbsp yoghurt; 1 tbsp lemon juice; 4 tbsp Natural Tree Syrup; 100g split almonds, lightly toasted.

Mix all the ingredients in a food processor and fill the pancakes. Fold into fours and serve with the Natural Tree Syrup & Banana Cream.

Natural Tree Syrup Fruit Smoothie

200g ripe fruit; juice of half a lemon; 200ml milk;
2 tbsp Natural Tree Syrup; 2 scoops vanilla ice-cream

Blend ingredients together in a mixer and serve with crushed ice.

Carrot and Natural Tree Syrup cake

4 egg yolks; 200ml Natural Tree Syrup; 200g grated carrot; juice and rind of lemon; pinch of cinnamon; 200g ground almonds; 80g wholemeal flour; 1 tsp powdered yeast; 4 egg whites; pinch of salt.

Mix the egg yolks and the syrup. Slowly add the rest of the ingredients except for the egg whites and the salt. Beat the egg white separately until stiff and add with a cutting mode. Bake in a pre-heated oven for 45 minutes at 180°.

Other tips:

Cold remedy:
Drink the Natural Tree Syrup with ginger, lemon and hot water.

Jet-lag
If you are going on a long-haul flight, follow the detox programme the day before you fly, the day you fly and the day after. Natural Tree Syrup will keep your stomach light and Japanese studies have reported the citric acid of the lemon being good for preventing blood clotting.

19: And finally

Rejuvenation, inner harmony and world peace

The world around us is a reflection of our thoughts, feelings and aspirations. The world is wanting in peace because we are wanting in peace. Only when we have inner harmony can we start sharing it. As long as we are confused in our minds, disturbed in our emotions and polluted in our physical bodies, it is impossible to achieve peace in our own being, and hence in the world around us.

One person may not be able to change the whole world, but we can all change a part of it – ourselves. By improving ourselves, we immediately make the world a better place. We diminish disharmony and increase peace. It's the best contribution we can make.

It works!

A flower: beautiful, fragrant, subtle, delicate, innocent, exquisite, pure. Do we ask how the flower blossoms?

Or do we simply appreciate, admire and adore the flower itself?

The human body is a miracle that functioned efficiently long before science came along. There are many theories on how the body works. Ayurvedic practitioners, naturopaths, herbalists, chiropractors, homoeopaths, kinesiologists, psychic healers and medical doctors all approach the body from a different perspective. There is truth in all the approaches. If someone were to take photographs of a mountain from many different angles, the photographs would all look different: yet they are all right, for the mountain is one and the same.

Similarly, there are many explanations of how and why this programme is so effective, whatever name you call it. Yet all the systems are compelled to agree with experience, which teaches one simple message: it works!

Seven maxims of rejuvenation

Be inspired. Remind yourself of all the positive reasons why you have chosen to embark in this program. Make a list. Remember **it is your choice,** and *you* will reap the benefits.

Be sensible. Follow closely the directions in this book.

Be strong. Abstain from eating or drinking anything other than the Natural Tree Syrup & lemon drink, occasional selected herb teas and citrus juices, laxative tea and pure water.

Be practical. Proper daily elimination is essential: consume plenty Natural Tree Syrup & lemon drink and use the laxative, salt water and skin brushing as additional aides.

Be wise. Remain active, physically and mentally. Exercise regularly but gently, pursue your favourite hobbies, explore new horizons, stay entertained.

Be careful. Ensure a soft landing in the transition back to regular eating by carefully following the directions when completing the programme.

Be happy. Remain cheerful throughout. You have to keep yourself company, so be fun to be with. Your happiness alone will brighten the world.

Useful contacts

For stockists of Natural Tree Syrup and other ingredients of *The Lemon Detox Diet*.

UK   www.lemondetox.com

UK & Eire Distributor
Pure Natural Products Ltd
P.O. Box 6554
Grantham
Lincs NG32 3FE

Tel: 0845 370 1012 Fax: 0845 370 1014
email: sales@purenaturalproducts.co.uk

USA   www.neerasupercleanse.com

USA Distributor
Supreme Joy Distributors
1298 Market Street
San Francisco, CA 94102
Tel: (888) 861-2798 or (415) 552-8245
email: info@neerasupercleanse.com

We'd like to hear how you enjoyed your chosen programme. Please send your thoughts, feelings and experiences to Pure Natural Products Ltd at the above address.

Natural Tree Syrup is manufactured by Puris AG, Switzerland.